Return to Sender

Michael S Hicks

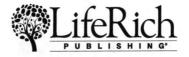

LifeRich Publishing is a registered trademark of
The Reader's Digest Association, Inc.

LifeRich Publishing books may be ordered
through booksellers or by contacting:

LifeRich Publishing
1663 Liberty Drive
Bloomington, IN 47403
www.liferichpublishing.com
1 (888) 238-8637

ISBN: 978-1-4897-2513-4 (sc)
ISBN: 978-1-4897-2512-7 (hc)
ISBN: 978-1-4897-2511-0 (e)

Library of Congress Control Number: 2019914854

Print information available on the last page.

LifeRich Publishing rev. date: 12/09/2019

The Childs Story

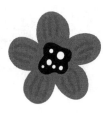

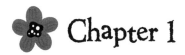 Chapter 1

"Hi," said the first voice I ever heard.

"Hi," I answered. "Where am I?"

"Your home."

"Where is home? What is home?" I said, still trying to figure out what was going on. All I knew before this was—well, nothing. Everything was so new, yet where I was now was where I always belonged.

"This is the place I first thought of you. See, I had a dream, and that dream was you, just as you are perfectly made. I created you to be with me forever, but there is something I need for you to do first," He said, further filling in the blanks of this puzzle that I was.

"Who are you?" was my next question, yet somehow I already knew, as a clock would know the time, as a leaf would know a breeze, as the fruit would know a branch. (Yet I knew I was about to be separated from this branch and fall into a place I didn't know.) My awareness of what was around me started to come into view. His words were hands, one pulling back the curtain and the other holding me as the newborn that I was. I could not describe this magnificent place, yet all around me was just the background to this person who held my every thought. Like the main character of a movie, I was made to play.

"Just call me PaPa. Some call me God, but let's keep it informal for now."

At the end of the statement came a name, a name I can't write down because there is no language that can write out its magnificence. The name hung out there in the air like a beautiful suit of clothes in a shopping window. All the while, I knew I would wear it one day, but not today. Still, I knew it was mine.

"I created you with a story in mind, and this story is entwined with many other stories. Its of a family started here where I had that dream, a dream of a family that will be with me forever," PaPa continued.

"What can I do, PaPa?" I said excitedly. I started to bounce up and down in His arms, ready to be a part of this fantastic story. I thought of all the brothers and sisters I would have, all the fun we would have in the beautiful fields I saw in the background of PaPa's face. Here, kernels of wheat were dancing while they were humming along to their favorite song sung by the gentle breeze. I started having my own dream, but it was not just mine. It was PaPa's, and I was just sharing it with Him. The trees scattered perfectly throughout the landscape stretching into the big sky, branching out to hold hands with one another. The sun played hide-and-seek behind the large branches, but there was no absence of light. So

I curiously followed the rays of light back to their source, and once again, I was face to face with PaPa. His smile was there ready to greet me, turning into a hug and the warmest kiss on my head.

Chapter 2

The suspense was aching in my soul to begin completing this dream I was a part of. I stared into PaPa's beautiful eyes to see water forming at the base of them. The water drops did not seem to belong there, so I reached out a wiped them away. Yet they kept coming. As I frantically wiped each one away, I felt this warm sensation in my own eyes. I stopped trying to hold back from Papas eyes what I could never keep up with only to reach out to my own to feel the same moisture dripping out.

"What are these, PaPa?" I said, holding out my finger.

"These are tears that I filled oceans with as I had to separate myself from my dream—a separation full of choices that I gave my dream. You will have these where I'm sending you." His conversation came back to my mind, the one where the sinking feeling came over me that I was the fruit picked from its place of conception to fall into the hands of someone I didn't know. PaPa reached out and wiped my tears first, revealing His beauty once again. "I have created you for so much, Jeremy."

Jeremy, I thought. *Who is that?*

"That's your name where you are going," PaPa explained.

He began telling me of all these plans He had for me. He spoke of how each part of me was magnificently made to accomplish His plan where we would be together forever. The more He talked of how I was made, the more excited I became. Just like a child seeing Disneyland in the distance after a trip that seemed like an eternity, I finally jumped out of His arms and ran around His legs to shed some of this excitement, all the while looking for the exit door.

He slowed me down with His words, and I finally stood looking up at Him with eyes filled with anticipation. Kneeling down, He gave me the last hug until we would meet again. It seemed to last forever with an intensity that said, "I'm sorry, but it's going to be okay." My arms felt limp from my return hug. I was ready to go.

Looking into my eyes with His one-of-a-kind smile, He said, "I love you. See you soon." His words told a story between the lines, a hidden knowledge that hurt Him deeply. He then reached up and closed my eyes.

Chapter 3

"Hello?" I said, recovering from what had just happened. All I remembered was PaPa closing my eyes and then this rush of warm air hitting me on both sides, seemingly from the afterthought of a man and women crashing into each other. I was in the middle of this decision they had made. The noise in the background of that moment was filled with laughter, excitement, passion, and curiosity, all in one explosive sound. Then it was quiet.

"Hello? PaPa?" I said again, receiving no reply. I felt as if I were swimming in this warm, dark pool, but I knew I was so small that someone would think I might not even be there.

"Hi, Jeremy," said a voice in the dark.

"PaPa, is that You?" I quickly asked. I felt so alone at that moment, not wanting to let this opportunity slip away, as I had just moments ago.

"Yes, it is," he replied. His voice gave me a picture in my mind of the warmest of smiles, so I quietly tucked it away for later, just in case.

"Why can't I see anything, PaPa?" I began to question.

"Jeremy, I'm in the process of knitting you together. Sit back while I create you in a way that will fit my amazing plans for you," He replied.

The excitement that had come the first time I heard this plan came back full force. This process was going on all around and inside of me, almost as if I were the process. Every movement echoed all His words, the same words that felt like hands. I noticed that His hands weren't holding me anymore; instead, they came in and around me as I was being put together. The whole time, there was a back-and-forth motion going on beneath me, as if I were in a cradle bringing me peace in this time of creation.

"PaPa, who is holding me?" I said, falling into this lullaby of movement.

"You're in your mother's womb. Do you remember the decision you were in the middle of? Well, that was where your mother met your father, and that is where your journey began," He replied.

"What's she like, PaPa? Does she know about me yet?" I said, all the while excitedly thinking a million different questions: what she looked like, what my dad would think of me, whether he would love me, what they liked to do, and on and on.

"She's amazing, Jeremy. I remember when I knitted her together in her mother's womb. I gave her the most beautiful eyes. You know what? I think I will give you her eyes. Your dad has an amazing personality, and I think I will give you that."

All His words made me think He was a painter, passionately pacing back and forth, pulling from this palette of endless colors. In a pouch on His side were grains of diamonds from a million different stars to build the frame of the masterpiece I was becoming. All His words started to muffle as I began to fall asleep in the rocking of an ocean all my own. As I slipped away, I slid through the front door of my first dream, the dream of what I would become and who would be there when I reached the other side.

Chapter 4

As I awoke, I stretched out my ... hmm, what were these? On the end of whatever they were, little sprouts wiggled at my command, so I used them to explore the rest of what I had become in what seemed like the blink of an eye.

Then I heard this chuckle from behind me.

"Those are arms," He answered. He continued His joyful explanation of each part I was discovering. I then started hearing voices from outside my cradle, but they were like a TV in a separate room. I reached up on what PaPa explained was a head to find the entry point of these new voices. When my hands fumbled upward, I felt their floppiness, so I started slapping them back and forth, laughing the whole time. In the middle of my fun, PaPa explained that they were called ears, and they gave me a way into this world around me I couldn't see yet.

I stopped playing with them, curious as to what was out there. It felt like I was spinning, with all these new noises surrounding me. I almost wanted to put these hands over them to filter out all these sounds that came in all at once. All the while, Papa was continuing His dance of creation while I was mesmerized at the first sound of her voice. Everything took a back seat to this orchestra that sounded like it was me talking yet was outside me. I think she just woke up, because I felt her stumble around, shaking up my ocean, which went with me, sloshing from one wall to another. Then I heard a door slam with a quick thump. Following that, it felt like her knees hit the ground, and sounds of agony came out.

Panicked, I called out to PaPa, "PaPa, is she okay?"

"She's fine Jeremy, but she's fixing to find out about you. That was kind of an alarm clock awakening her to the fact that someone else is here," He said with another chuckle.

PaPa just went right back to the canvas, joyfully putting me together. I went back to my listening, putting my ear to the wall of my new home. I heard a jingling, then a door close. We were moving pretty fast, so I guessed we were going somewhere important. Soon we were there, and they called her into a room. The voices were unclear, but I was well aware of the nervousness my mother felt as she went into this room. I felt her lie down as another person talked in the background, explaining what they were doing. She jumped a little as something touched her belly. Then whatever it was started rolling over my head as if I were on a copy machine. I felt like I was on stage and the spotlight was on me, swinging back and forth over my head.

Then came the news of my coming-out party! I was so happy to hear her excitement about this new family. I jumped a little, splashing around in my warm ocean, then settled down to listen to her reaction. The other voice delivered the news, and then there was a very long pause. The silence was followed by a quiet "thank you" as she got off the table. Then the other voice stopped her as she was leaving the room, handing her something, saying, "Here's another option." I had never had the privilege of hearing something that clear. It came as a gift, in the form of a forewarning of an option I would have never chosen.

Chapter 5

It seemed as if an earthquake started as she closed the car door. Then the tears came as she caressed me through her belly, all the while sobbing the words "What are we going to do?"

I remembered the tears PaPa cried when he told me I would soon know their meaning. I joined her in her grief, all the while wanting to hold her to let her know it was going to be all right. Still, this feeling, which I had never felt before, became its own earthquake inside my chest. I heard in the break between the convulsions of sadness a broken conversation with PaPa just saying the words, *Please help me. Please help me. I need You.* She never said PaPa's name, but I knew who she was talking to because His voice was who I would cry out to. I simply cried with her, telling her, "I need you too."

As I was fixing to call out to PaPa myself, I heard a ringing sound coming from around her waist. Startled, she cleared her throat, answering the sound. I could tell she was frustrated, as the conversation started with a soft tone, then erupted with yelling.

"This is all your fault!"

I wondered if she was talking about me, but I shook it off, remembering all PaPa had planned for me. Slamming something against the dashboard the force of her driving off pushed me to the back of my home, as she serenaded me with this loud music she knew by heart. Every turn threw me back and forth, making me a little nervous, wondering where this place was that she needed to be so quickly.

My head hit the front as she quickly stopped, followed by the slamming of a door. After a brisk walk, she banged on a door like she was the cops, bringing out a familiar voice. The frustration came back as if she was still in the car, letting this person have it with everything she had. Then my curiosity was cured when she made the statement: "Well, you're the father!"

She said it with a mixture of anger and desperation so he would take on this decision they both made.

Is it true? Is this my daddy? I cried out in my head, forgetting the tone of the room. I got all excited listening for just a word from my daddy! Though it would be my daddy here, he was still a part of me too. In between the screams and flying objects that didn't really affect me came the most tremendous blow of all.

"The kid's not mine. It's your fault," he yelled back.

Silence filled the air, filled this womb, actually, my whole universe, while the stars and I waited for a statement that would fix what had just happened. As the moments passed, gravity seemed to multiply. With no words came the reality I did not want to face. Papa was wrong. I was a mistake.

Chapter 6

This next ride was a lot slower, without the loud music, without tears, just silence.

I wish she could hear me was all I could think as I banged on these walls with my tiny arms, just to let her know I was here. I just didn't want her to forget what I knew I was going to be. I didn't want to be rejected again. I didn't want ... to not be known. I guess that's the way she felt too. I felt the same intensity banging on my walls as she was banging on that door. She knew, as I did, that on the other side was someone who was now a part of her, the part that would make all this possible, even though she hadn't asked for it. Just like me. I hadn't asked for this, but I knew what I wanted: I wanted to live. I wanted to be a part of this grand story PaPa told me.

I turned to this picture of PaPa's studio in my head, asking, "PaPa, are You still here?"

"Yes, Jeremy. I'm right here," He replied, giving me a room to breathe that breath I had been holding in since I heard I was a mistake.

"PaPa, am I a mistake? Is there something wrong with me?" I asked, trying to make sense of all this.

"No, Jeremy, you are perfectly made. There's not a thing wrong with you," He replied, bringing me some comfort, comfort I wanted to share with my mom.

I continued to drill PaPa with all these questions crowding my head: "Why did my daddy reject me? Why did Mom not answer my knock? What's going to happen to me, PaPa?"

I could tell from PaPa's tone that He was sad too, but at the same time he was struggling as if His hands were tied.

"Jeremy, I gave my creation a choice, a choice made by them, not me. I don't always agree with their choice, but I love them, so I give them this gift. At the same time, I am here when they call. When your mom called to me earlier, I sent an answer, but ultimately, it is her choice."

"Where's my choice, Papa!"

I screamed so loud I think my mom heard it, because she got real quiet.

"It's okay."

I listened to my mom comfort me, but I screamed again in my anger, "My name is Jeremy. Call me by my name. Make me real!"

She continued to comfort me as a problem with no name.

PaPa interrupted, "Jeremy, she is hurting, and you are real, more real than you could ever imagine," he replied in her defense. "I chose you, Jeremy. Remember that above all. My plans won't change. Only the decisions I gave as a gift will."

I thought about what PaPa said, all the while knowing He loved me better than anyone ever could. My thoughts started breaking down in this cradle, where I felt Mom rocking me as she cried once again out to PaPa. A soft song eased its way through the sobs that spoke directly to my heart. One more song she knew by heart because someone sang it to her. Each note seemed to squeeze me a little more, letting me know she loved me. I was finally able to release this thought of never being known, which helped me fall asleep. But I still didn't have a name.

Chapter 7

I woke up to the shuffling of papers flying about at a crazy pace. Mom's voice was frantic as she tried to see how all this was going to work out. She was talking to herself as if she were a calculator putting numbers in the air, matching them with weightier numbers. What started as sighs became screams.

That ringing sound came once again from around her waist. Then, throwing her papers down frustrated, she answered it. With a gruff tone, she answered as if to tell the other person, *Unless you have some money to give me, you have no business talking to me.* She softened as she said the words "Hi, Momma." Her feet started to shuffle like the guy hustling on the streets, asking you which cup your money is under. I wondered if she would talk about me making me real to this world I longed to see. She bounced around in conversation with this game of keep-away until she was finally cornered into revealing the truth. I could tell from the answers she gave that no matter what revelations her mother gave her, she could not see it. I guess it was an answer to her prayer, just not in the way she pictured it.

I stretched out my arms, yawning, ready to start my day, but Mom wasn't. She was done talking to her mother and now was crawling back in bed, throwing the covers over her head. The gentle shaking of a broken person steadily rippled through my home. Then, wiping her tears, she slowly sat up in the bed and grabbed a piece of paper off the table. I heard her dial a number slowly, then hang up, then hang up again, then again, then again. After all these tries, this time, she waited for someone to answer. Soon I hear a person on the opposite end giving her information about times and places.

I was kind of worried now if she was all right, so I called out, "PaPa, can you let her know it's okay?"

His trustworthy voice replied, "Jeremy, I sent her mother to talk to her. I can only give direction. She has to make the decision. But I will keep trying"

What decision, I thought? I just shrugged it off, thinking the best I could at this moment, having faith in PaPa. The sound of keys jingling floated like wind chimes to my ears, making me wonder where we were going.

Heaviness surrounded us like a man walking up to a noose made for him. The car started but idled for the longest. Then, just like the phone call, the car started. It was turned off more than once. All the while, it was as if she was listening to PaPa in those brief moments between decisions. I felt this fight going on inside of her all the while in her heart, protecting me, then letting me go because I was too heavy. Then the decision to keep going won, and we started to drive.

❀ Chapter 8

The longest trip of my life was now in motion, trotting along like a funeral procession. I was waiting for some kind of noise to take my mind off what I knew was about to happen, but I was blind too, as if my eyes had not been given freedom. I heard her roll the window down so she could breathe in deep, then let the breeze wipe away from her mind where she was going. We pulled into the parking lot and sat there longer than we had to. The ringing sound came again, but she stopped it, again, again, and again. I wanted to answer it for her, 'cause I knew PaPa was on the other line.

With a deep sigh, she stepped out of the car, and we headed to our destination. As we got closer to the door, someone stopped her with the kindness voice, asking her to talk. Mom stood there for a few minutes. Then tears started to fall like anchors from a ship holding it in port. Mom sat down while this person presented her with other options, just like that lady had in the doctor's office, except this one was better for me. After some time talking, Mom got up, and I thought she had listened, but

I felt her continue in the first direction. I felt so stuck not being able to sit down and talk with her myself, to tell her of this beautiful plan she would be a part of because I was the key to it. I'd heard it, and I knew it was real, just like me.

The doors must have been heavy, since she had to grunt with effort to open them. Coldness started to creep into my home, taking away any warmth that was there before. She talked to someone, then started filling out some paperwork, stopping over and over again as I felt her look at the door she just came in.

Someone called her name, and she went with them. Every step she made was into what seemed like a big freezer. I huddled in the corner of my home as she crawled up onto an even colder table. There was one more moment of silence as she waited, which was one more chance I wish she would use to leave this cold place.

Without warning, I felt PaPa hold my hand, as a father would when his child had to walk into a dark room. When I asked Him what was going on, He just stayed silent. I swiveled my head all around, trying to find something else to hold onto, only to find even PaPa's studio was no more. All forms of security were gone in this moment except PaPa's hand, which still felt like a big jacket on a kids coat hanger, ready to let me go to. Then someone came into the room, giving orders to others. Then he got so close to me, I could smell the lunch he had just finished. I would have closed my eyes, but they had not been open here on this side of life, yet I still wanted to cover them. PaPa's grip became more secure the closer this stranger got. His hand felt restrained, but it remained right where it was supposed to be, never letting me go. Then I felt His words right in my new ears: "See you soon."

Soon, I thought, *What about now? What about this amazing plan? What about.* Suddenly, I was distracted by a cold metal object grabbing my foot. I felt Mom grab the handles of the bed, clenching from the pain, or maybe she felt mine. I joined in by grabbing PaPa even tighter. The pulling from the object became so painful I screamed!

"Momma, Momma, please protect me!"

The object started tearing away all PaPa had created. Yet as I tried to fight, screaming at it to stop, I saw I was no match for this instrument, which knew no conscious or the voice I had. I couldn't take it anymore. Still, I tried squeezing PaPa's hand even more, holding on, thinking this was a mistake, just as my daddy said. A horrible sound that reminded me of when Mom was cleaning the house came closer and closer, taking ahold of me

"No, no, no."

Then it was dark.

Chapter 9

"Hi" was the voice I heard next. Now seeing I could open my eyes, I peeked with just one of them, in case it was a trick. In front of me was the beautiful field I had seen behind PaPa during my first conversation. Opening the other eye, I saw a little guy like me standing there with the biggest smile.

"HI, my name is Bobby," he continued. "It's okay. You're safe now."

My eyes adjusted to my new surroundings, bringing into view the dancing grains of wheat all around me. Each stalk reached out to me, tickling me, trying to get me to laugh, as if to let me know, *It's all right now.* After the tickle fest, Bobby gave me the biggest hug I ever had. Well, not the biggest. PaPa was the best at that. The stalks of wheat all around me did the same, surrounding me with gentle little hands, holding me while they rocked me back and forth as the breeze kissed my ears with their beautiful song. All these emotions came on me like a puppy running up its master's leg, making me laugh and cry at the same time. Then all the memories came, one by one: Mom's voice, Dad's rejection, the cold room, my new hands, and the ears I played with for the first time came out like one of those old Polaroid cameras that produced pictures instantly. As each moment came out, they suddenly grew wings, flying off into that endless blue sky, never to return.

When the last one was nothing but a dot in the sky, my mind was now a blank slate, ready to write down all that I had seen around me, because everything now was right. My eyes, like a pen, started drawing on this blank slate a joy I could not describe. I wish I could tell you more, but it's indescribably beautiful. My new family is running and hiding in the wheat fields as the stalks help out by covering them up while they play hide-and-seek. The trees reach down, picking them up, setting them on their branches, allowing them to climb to a height that never ends. Laughter crowds the air like a dance floor, staying in rhythm with the songs sung by the breeze.

Then I saw Him, PaPa.

Quickly forgetting Bobby and all my new friends, I started to run. I never ran so hard, actually. *Hmmm, I've never run,* I thought as I giggled fitting in with all this laughter. As I tore through this path from me to the other part of me, the stalks split right down the middle, giving a clear shot to the one I love. There at the end of this journey, I tackled PaPa knocking Him down in the field with my joy. We laughed so hard, as if it would never end, as we rolled around on the field of His dream. Holding me in the air, He stood up, putting me on His shoulders. Then he said the words that started eternity: "Welcome home, my child."

The Mothers Story

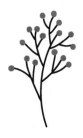

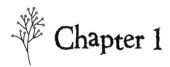 # Chapter 1

It was like any other day that I had tried to live before, except with a twist. I had come home from college for a visit waking up in my old room after a great day with my family, who had taken me to church even though I'm not into that kind of thing. It was always a great memory for me that I hadn't had a chance to live in a while: how we would go to church, then out to eat, followed by a great Sunday nap. We would always seem to wake up at the same time without an alarm. Then, after eating leftovers, we took a vote for a movie or games. Games seemed to win consistently, even though, like church, I wasn't really into it. But it was family, and you take whatever just to be with them.

I used to believe in this Jesus thing when I was younger, going to youth group and camps. I would listen to Christian music, pray to this someone who heroically sent His son to save me, and give my money to the Church. I do have to say, it felt like I knew PaPa (that's what I used to call him) and He knew me. Then, one day, at sixteen, I came home to a roomful of people. Uniforms crowded around my mom, and they were all leaning over my dad, lying there face up on the floor. His rosy cheeks were now cold stones, his hands laid by his side instead of wrapped around my mom or holding her hand. He was the strong one who held me when I had my heart broken the first time, the one who led the family in prayer every night in a home I could count on because he was always there.

I stood there as an outside observer since everyone was fixed on my dad, giving the rest of the room to my mother, who was crying and praying for this not to be true. Slowly the uniforms drifted by me as I stood like the painting by the front door, which people knew was there and thought was pretty but never said so. Forced smiles flashed my direction, like the ones I gave when I didn't know what to say to the homeless man I passed on the sidewalk.

Trying to snap out of my daze, I joined my mom on the living room floor, jumping straight into God's words. We stayed there where time stood still, just praying, believing, and not giving up. My mind wandered back to this dream I thought I was in, telling PaPa how good he was, and I knew he wouldn't let anything like this happen to a family that loved him so much. Still, he lay there lifeless as the EMTs urged us to let them take him away. Swinging at them to stay away, my mom put her hands on my shoulders, softly crying. And that's where it happened, the place I knew this god thing was just a prop.

See, my dad was my hero, the model of what a man

should be. As much as I protested, my dad was always taking hold of my mom, smooching her in the kitchen, in the car, or in the middle of Walmart, telling her how beautiful she was. He would take me to the movies and even concerts that played music I knew he couldn't stand. Yet he never let on and danced right along with me in the car on the way. When he was wrong, he was the first one to admit it. But he never changed his mind when it came to what was best for our family.

I curled up next to my mom watching the movie that had won out this time because Dad used to be the tiebreaker, and he loved the games. I slowly drifted as my mom caressed my hair while that feeling rushed over me. The one that I hadn't felt since before the day God took my dad away. Once again it felt like it should have,home.

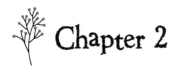 Chapter 2

I woke up to my mom shaking me so hard I almost fell off the couch where she had stealthfully left me the night before.

"You're gonna miss you flight, honey. Let's go!" came the words that woke me from the dream of my knight in shining armor, coming to rescue me. Getting my feet tangled up in my grandma's blanket she had brought from my room to cover me, I hit the floor. My mom broke into laughter as I sheepishly grinned on my way back up to the shower to get ready. Everything was pretty much packed up, with all my laundry clean from this mighty woman I called Mom, my other hero and the one who never wavered from her belief in God's plan in our tragedy. At the same time, in my wandering, she never gave up on me, never changed her love for me, and never stopped praying for me (she always reminded me of that). I watched her grab all my bags, putting them by the front door so I didn't miss a thing as I threw on my beanie so I didn't have to do my hair.

I saw her start to tear up by the painting at the

front door, never breaking from her task. I reached out, grabbing her away from what could be done another time to hug her in a time that needed to be now. She almost broke in my arms as I hugged her so hard, telling her I was strong now and that I loved her more than words could say. Shaking it off, seeing the Uber show up, I ran out with what I had while she stood at the front door. I knew she wanted to take me. Really, she wanted to keep me, but she loved me enough to let me go and make a life of my own.

Before putting on my seatbelt, I made the back windshield of the Uber the front by turning around, waving the whole time until she was no more. Quickly switching from one world to another, I pulled out my phone and started to text my best friend from college, Sheila. Quickly she replied with all her crazy emojis—of unicorns and happy faces—which was her quick way of jumping up and down, telling me she was ready for me to come back. We had been roommates for these first two years of college, and she was the person I always wanted to be, carefree and bold. She had introduced me to the other side of life, where no rules were applied. There, I could cover up all the brokenness that remained after that fateful day.

Getting to the airport just in time, I checked in, watching all the other college students heading back from holidays. Some I had seen on campus. Some I had never seen before. Yet we were all in the same mode of escape, flying away to a place we could leave all we had been taught to learn a whole new way. No restrictions held us down, and the possibilities were endless – and so were the mistakes we could make. Even though my family had never really judged me when I decided to step away from the whole God thing, the church stood ready to take their place. All the people who used to be my friends from church took a step back from me instead of walking with me; I guess they were afraid my decision would rub off on them. I used to wait for them to call me in my battle of conscience and faith, but I just faded away from their concern, like that painting by the front door. That painting was done by my dad. It was the most beautiful collection of colors and images that only he could explain, and even though it was by the front door, it was the center of my heart. I guess I disappeared from the church, yet there I remained, just like my dad's painting, whose meaning only I knew.

Continuing to think about all these things, I looked out the window, watching everything I had known for so long become smaller, just like my mom, just like me to this town, the Church, and God.

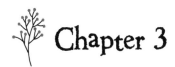

Chapter 3

We hit the runway with a sudden jolt of force shaking me like my mom did this morning. Just then, I kinda freaked out a little. I must have been so deep in sleep. I think that's because I was having the grandest dream of my little boy with thousands of people around him intently, listening like he had the answer to something they had been searching for for so long. I think he was my child. The connection I had with him was one of a kind. Shaking it off because it was so real, I got into the rat race of getting out of the plane and getting my luggage so I could breathe my own air again.

Getting to the arrival area, there she was, my best friend, Shelia, all decked out in party gear and the car filled with a bunch of people I didn't know. She threw her arms around me. Then, after throwing my bags in the trunk of her hooptie, which we affectional called the Gray Bomber, she quickly explained that there was a coming-home party for everyone at college returning from the holidays. Shelia was never one to miss a party, and even if I didn't want to, she always got me to go. However, there were times when I just needed some quiet, a place to see where I was and where I wanted to be, only to get irritated every time, since these two never lined up. It was like trying to fit a piece from another puzzle into the one I was working on. I could keep trying a million different ways, but it would never fit. Maybe I could cut it to fit, but in the end, the whole puzzle would be off.

In those times, I still thought of PaPa in heaven and how I would like to see him one day, how my daddy was there to hold my grandma and all those who had come before me in my family, who believed. That eternal tug never left me, but tonight, I was gonna drown it out, just like a kid whose parents took off and left the house to them. We all started singing to the song of the moment while we passed around the bottle. I don't even know what it was, but it tasted like cinnamon, and I knew it would take me away from where I was right now, at least in my mind.

We got to the party, jumping out in unison, screaming as if we had just discovered the promise land after a long trip. The lights coming from the front door moved in rhythm to the pounding beat, becoming a dance partner that only I could see. The room was chaos, controlled only by these walls surrounding us. I continued to flow in and out of the crowd, with Sheila dancing as we went. Soon we were joined by the jocks, who saw an easy target, but we shoved them off, laughing as we continued exploring.

After a while of drinking and dancing, we found

ourselves on the back porch, and there he was, this six-foot gorgeous guy with a man bun and the body of a Greek god. Shelia and I looked at each other with the silent OMG. Then she pushed me over his way. Falling right into his beer, I kinda laughed, like I did after my feet got tangled up in Grandma's blanket. That thought raised the question of whether I should even be here. That was broken by his tenor voice and smooth words. He was so nice, and I was so drunk that conversation soon turned into making out. The rest of the night was kind of a blur. Spots of colors hit the canvas of my mind but not enough to complete the picture of what happened.

The next morning, I woke up in his bed, feeling like my head weighed a thousand pounds. He was still sleeping, and I was just ready to leave. I texted Sheila to find she was there too. I threw my clothes on and met her at the front of his fraternity. We drove away silently, turning down the music, which had been so loud last night. I just sat there looking out the window as Shelia drove us to our apartment. My mind raced around in itself, trying to pick up the pieces of what I thought was just an escape, but something inside me said it had been so much more.

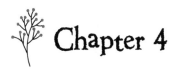

Chapter 4

The next month and a half flew by with school and the usual drama of life. Shelia left college. She would try again next year. She had pushed the boundaries, only to find failing grades waiting for her when she broke through to the other side. The house was as quiet as I sometimes wished it would be, but now it was quiet all the time, leaving me with only my schoolwork and my thoughts.

I woke up one morning after that same dream again of the boy and all those people hanging on his every word. I had a sickening feeling. Yelling out an OMG, I ran to the bathroom, holding my mouth so I wouldn't drop last night's food on the floor. My knees hit the ground, where I deposited everything from the night before. I hung there for a few more minutes. Then my mind started to race. First, the sensible reasons. It was a virus or food poisoning. But the one that made me nervous was still outside, knocking on the door of my heart. That night of escape came rushing back, hitting me over and over again just like someone tapping me on my shoulder, trying to hand me something I had dropped. Except I just wanted to walk away, because I didn't want that. That was not in my plans for my future. Not like this. Not this way. Not right now.

I headed out the door to get the first appointment possible with my doctor. Grabbing my keys, I rushed out the door and into the car. Shelia had left it for me to use while she was gone. Actually, it probably wouldn't have made it on a long trip anyway. They had an open schedule, so I was brought straight in. Sitting in that room, I felt a breeze of reality blow in by my surroundings. Pictures of pregnancy were on the walls, not making it any easier to ignore the possibility I don't even have to mention, because somehow I knew.

The doctor came in with the regular questions. Finally coming to the conclusion of pregnancy, they ran some tests. She came back in, giving me the news I already knew. I think I knew the next day. Laying me back on the table, they did a sonogram, lathering my belly up with that cold gel, making me jump, then running the machine back and forth to reveal my new guest. A tear crept out like the first signs of a broken pipe, so I reached up to wipe it away and mentally put some tape on it until I got in the car. I quietly said, "Thank you" and headed to the door, feeling so lost in how I was going to handle it. I think the doctor saw the look. She stopped me at the door and handed me a pamphlet showing me places I could have an abortion. I quietly tucked it in my purse, just trying to be polite. I could never do that. At least I didn't think so.

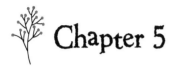

Chapter 5

I exploded like a rain cloud locked up for too long. Violently I shook as I caressed my belly, talking to what I could no longer deny.

"What are we doing to do?" were the words I said to what I couldn't see, followed by the words to the other one I could not see, PaPa.

"Please, help me. Please, help me. I need You" came blubbering out in small doses. In the middle of it all, I felt my phone ringing in my pocket. Pulling it out and seeing who it was startled me. It was the Greek god guy I had hooked up with. I had been lonely one night after a bottle of wine, so I texted him. I guess he finally got it, or he was now just answering. I tossed the idea of telling him back and forth. He needed to know. He needed to take responsibility for his part in this.

I cleared my throat and wiped my tears, giving me an unclouded view to answer the phone. I started off with the pleasantries of "Hi" and "How have you been doing?" His smooth voice made me smile, giving me a sort of permission to tell him the news. After a few more sentences, he asked where I was, and I used that as the front door to let him know about this situation. I went in with the belief that there would be some intelligent banter and we could work this out. When I told him the news, there was a quiet streak that went on too long, so I asked if he was still there. His voice changed as if I had accused him of something wrong. He asked questions like "Who else have you slept with?" and "Are you sure it's mine?" He was pushing away, just like I had when I first thought of it, so I tried to calm him down, but it didn't work. Then I started in on him, escalating what I thought was going to be a normal conversation into a yelling match. We played hot potato with the subject until I heard a click, then silence. Not the kind earlier where it was just silent, but this Idiot just hung up on me.

I yelled, "Oh hell, no!" slamming my phone into the dashboard, shattering the screen and any hope of using it again. My backup phone was tucked away somewhere in my drawer by my bed, so I put the car in drive and turned the radio on full blast, taking me back to the day I came home from holidays. Speeding off, I screamed out the song by heart all the way to his frat house.

Getting out, I slammed the car door, then headed up the porch, barging my way in and up the stairs to his door, knocking on the top like the cops do to let him know I wasn't going anywhere. He answered the door, and I immediately started off the conversation where he had ended it by hanging up. He tried to talk, but I didn't let him. I was the one in control of this *Jerry Springer Show* on his front doorstep.

Finally, it came down to the nail in the coffin, as I said, "Well, you're the father!"

He shot back with words that sent a shock through me, landing right in my stomach. "The kid's not mine. It's your fault."

I stood there looking at him with nothing to say. After a few seconds of him looking at my blank stare, he slammed the door in my face. My knees started to hurt from the weight of my heart. Where was my daddy right now? Where was PaPa? This was all I could think, but I knew I had done this, just like he said. Why would either one of them want to talk to me? I slumped away, defeated, lost, and numb. My whole world was crashing around me as I made my way back to the car and started home. All I could think was *How could this happen to me?*

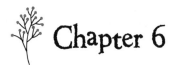

Chapter 6

The longest ride of my life was now challenged by this one, the first being coming back from the funeral of my daddy. I remember it as if it were yesterday, with the winter air in my face as I looked out at his gravesite, waiting for a miracle, just like I was right now. Doing the same as I did that day, I had the window down with the sun on my face and the cold wind reminding me of winter. I'd made this a thing since the day of Dad's funeral. It was my way of clearing my mind to wipe away all the confusion that made me want to end it all. I hadn't felt depression like I did right then in a long time. It all started the day God didn't come through by bringing back my dad. That day, I walked away from what might have been there, but now reality took his place.

I stared out the window as numb as my face was from the cold air, shuffling back and forth this hot potato that was mine and mine alone. It never cooled down long enough for me to digest it. I pulled into the nearest parking lot I saw, feeling nauseated, tumbling out the door as I had at the toilet earlier today. As I leaned over,

I felt a small knocking coming from my stomach, like it was trying to talk to me. This is a conversation I did not want to have, but judging by its persistence, it did.

The word "it" started to annoy me, but I didn't want a name attached, because then this would be real. I tried to hold onto the same illusion as when I looked out the window one more time, believing for a miracle. I closed the door, sitting there, just wanting to stay in this moment so I didn't have to deal with the next one. Yet I knew I had to get home.

I opened the door to my apartment and just stood there imagining my friend Shelia was there. Then it switched to coming home and my family waiting for me in the foyer, just like the day I came home, where the unveiling of Dad's painting awaited me. The older I'd gotten, the more I understood its complex structure of textured colors: some were bright, some were dull, and some just looked as if they didn't belong, just like the situation I was in. Still, when Daddy explained it, he said it was a metaphor for life – how all these different situations make a beautiful masterpiece. I don't know how he was so proud of that painting; it didn't fit the definition of any landscape, person, or object that you could go up to and say, "Hey, that looks like a car or house." Still, when he looked at it, he glowed, just like when he looked at Mom, or when he looked at me.

I made my way in, throwing everything down without my usual type-A–personality organizing, controlling every piece around me. I saw no use to it, because I now had something I couldn't control. I crawled into bed, leaning against the headboard, staring at my belly, covering it with tears I couldn't control. Maybe it was the hormones; perhaps it was the fact that I was a failure, that color of failurie which now messed up this masterpiece of mine showing me how things should be I'm kind of glad my dad wasn't alive, because I couldn't tell him that his little girl got knocked up.

I'm such a failure. How can I bring this life into the world with such a screwed-up mom. Think of all the problems it would have right off the bat. It wouldn't have a dad, it would have an immature mother, and this world is just screwed up with all its wars, political stupidity, and uncertainties.

I slowed down and started to quiet my mind from going through all the pros and cons of this situation by closing my eyes, but not tightly enough to stop the tears. Then I drifted back to when I was a child and this tune my mom made for me that put me to sleep, a song that made all the monsters go away, giving me a sense of peace. It came out of me without even thinking, so I pointed its words towards this life that was inside me, rocking back and forth the child that was mine but which I would not name.

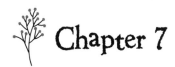 # Chapter 7

I woke up with a purpose. I was determined I was going to figure this out. My type-A personality took back control, starting this frantic shuffling of school papers, bills, and calculations of the cost of this life. I put down all that would need to happen in this process, tackling this issue with analytical fervor. It didn't take long for me to run out of numbers and ways that would explain how this was going to happen. I finally just threw it all up in the air, screaming out my inability with such clarity there was no denying it.

Then I heard my phone ringing from my jacket hanging from the kitchen chair I was sitting at, the throne to my war room that had lost. It startled me, because I never thought this thing would ever work again. I looked to see who it was, but I couldn't tell since the screen was busted, so I gave an irritated grunt, thinking this better be Publishers Clearing House and not a telemarketer. When I answered it, I heard my mom's sweet voice on the other end. I loved her voice; it took me back to the song she used to sing me, making me feel safe. The words of encouragement always showered on me, but today, I didn't deserve that voice.

We started the back and forth of a mother-daughter talk, asking me how I'd been doing, how school was, what I'd been up to. This time there was a tone of suspiciousness in Mom's questions, as if she knew something. Finally, she told me that the Lord had put me on her heart, telling her that I needed her. I tried my best to keep the truth from her, but I couldn't. Like a tractor beam, she pulled me in with that connection only a mother and daughter have. Then, just like a bag of groceries falling off the kitchen counter, out came the secrets I had been keeping, except some of the items had been in there too long and were rotten.

After my kitchen turned into a confessional, I wished she was like a priest: she'd give me a few Hail Mary's and Mother May I's, or whatever it was, and then it would all be over. Instead, she poured out no judgment, even though I wished she would have—then I could have agreed with her—but only words of wisdom and concern. I fought her at every turn, telling her I had already thought of that. She offered for me to come home, but I was my own woman, and I made my own decisions. I wasn't a kid anymore was the attitude I gave that offer. Finally, she gave me space and asked me to think about what we had talked about it.

Hanging up, I ran to my room to get back under the covers, trying to hide from the decision I had to make.

The tears showed up again, telling me of one more thing I couldn't control. I'd had enough. I just had to do it. I just had to give in. I just had to make the call. I sat up in bed, grabbing the pamphlet from the nightstand. Grabbing the house phone right beside it, I dialed the numbers, hearing the answering service that took the place of humans giving me options. Quickly I hung up, then reached out one more, trying to make it through the whole process, but I hung up again. After a few more tries, I got a human voice, giving me the open schedule that I could fill right now. I confirmed and headed straight for the door, grabbing the keys to the car.

Once in the car, I started it right up, then shut it off, trying to decide what I had already decided on. Trying again, I gave another few pauses to what I had talked myself into. Then, on the last turn of the key, I went straight for the gearshift, forcing it down like the gavel on a judge's bench, and I started to drive.

Chapter 8

The cold breeze was hitting me from my rolled-down window, feeding me fresh air to blow out any thought of going back. I went back to my debate club from high school in my mind, remembering it was my favorite class. No one could come against me with their weak ideas, so full of holes. I would stop them in any direction they came from, taking them down like a WWE wrestler. My viciousness was known throughout these juvenile halls, but now I was in a debate I didn't want to be in, one against myself, against another life, against what I believed myself. Now the logic was my foe in this debate, creating an atmosphere of decision that carried a weight I could not handle, so I just ended it. I wouldn't allow any more discussion, dropping my gavel just like the gearshift earlier, setting me in the direction of what had to be done. It just made sense. I was just tired of running back and forth from each table to defend what I had just shot down.

Finally, we arrived in the parking lot. I stopped for a moment, remembering what I just said: *we*. To know something or someone so intimately has never been an issue. No boyfriend, friend, family member, not even my dad, could fill this place inside me. The thought of coming back to this car with it being just me took my breath away, like coming around a hallway corner and running into someone who knocks the breath out of you. As I took my breath back from the frozen air around me, it helped to take away any warmth that would take me away from my mission.

The ringing came just as I was about to step from the car. I knew it was my mom; I just had that feeling. Looking at it for a minute, I rejected the call. Once again it rang, then again and again and again. Each time, I denied what I knew: I should answer. She seemed to be taking the place in the opposite side of this debate that I had shut down, and with every rejection of her call my gavel once again shut down any argument against what I had decided. Finally, I just threw the phone down in the floorboard of the passenger seat and slammed the door, but the one thing I couldn't leave was this life inside of me.

I briskly walked to the clinic, keeping my eye on the door so as not to be distracted again. Then a voice from what seemed heaven pierced the wall I had put around me. Stopping in my tracks, I turned to see an elderly woman sitting on a bench close to the entrance. Somehow, I knew she was there to talk me out of this. It was as if God kept trying to stop me, but in my stubbornness, I remembered the choice He had also in bringing my daddy back to me.

The funny thing was she didn't have a protest sign. Nor was she yelling at me from some self-righteous platform. Instead, she was just there and available. After her introduction, the women on the bench asked to share a story with me, skipping the questions of "What are you doing here?" which I had an answer for, but with this approach, I didn't. I sat beside her, giving her the floor in this last debate, which wasn't a debate, but as I listened, it became a testimony of a decision she had made to enter a similar door. Soon the tears finally broke through this wall I had built up, just as her voice did. She simply held me, offering no advice or reminders of what I had done or could do. All the while, I felt two knocks coming from inside me, one in my heart, the other in my womb.

Then came all the tasks that would come with deciding not to go through with it, how the dad didn't want it, how it would suffer from my own instability, how, how, how, how? So I just politely said, "Thank you" and continued my journey in. As I gave a quick glance back, I saw her sitting there with tears falling from her eyes, looking like diamonds, as if God himself sat there waiting on me, but I turned away.

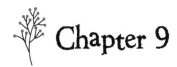

Chapter 9

Stepping up to the entrance, I realized this was the heaviest door I had ever tried to open. As I stepped in, the lady at the widow gave me some paperwork to fill out, so I made a place unconsciously closest to the door, looking back, waiting on someone to come in and save me. Maybe the dad would come running in, telling me to stop and that he loved me, reassuring me that we could live happily ever after, because this is the way it's supposed to be, right? This is the way it played out in the movies. This is how I was raised. This is the checklist on the paper labeled, "The Perfect Life." But this wasn't.

Finishing the paperwork, I handed it in, and before I had a chance to sit back down, they called me to the back. It was like walking into a freezer the further back I went. We reached the room where the nurse directed me to the table and started preparing for the procedure. As she finished up, the doctor came into the place with a bedside manner that made me feel like a fast-food customer. I could tell he'd just had lunch, because I could smell the salami radiating throughout the room. As he started, he let me know to just relax. How the hell am I supposed to relax? I felt as he pulled from inside me pieces of what was once whole shooting pain, deep within my womb and soul. I grabbed the sides of the bed from the pain. All the while in my mind, I wanted to use them to stop him. I wanted to push him away, because every moment that passed was my chance to save him, my baby. I couldn't say anything because I knew it was too late. The final step was now in place as I felt an emptying going on inside me from the vacuum pulling out all hope of ever going back. I screamed in my head as reality came to close for me. Then I exploded with the regret of someone who once had a choice.

The doctor quietly left, leaving the nurses to explain how I was going to be taken into a room and that I should wait for thirty minutes, and then I could leave. When we got into the recovery room, there was a row of women who had just made the same decision. I think if there was ever a sound that would come from hell, it was here. Their wails bounced off the walls, punching me in my already wounded soul. Knowing they couldn't keep me, I just walked out. There was no way they were going to keep me here in this hell.

I walked out of the clinic with all those same voices that told me to do it now condemning me for killing my child. With my head down, I made my way back to my car, once again passing the same women who had loved me before. I heard that same voice of love, with no words, stand from that bench and become the very arms of what God would feel like. I collapsed into the void of any strength of my on as she held me, crying in unison. It was as if this stranger was living her own decision all over again. Lowering me onto the bench, I leaned into her chest as she caressed my hair.

Even though the tears continued, my soul was comforted enough to say, "I'm sorry. I'm sorry!" but she just quieted me, reminding me, "It's okay. God still loves you."

"How could He love a murder?" I mumbled through the excess.

Then all the things I knew before of PaPa came flooding back—of His unchanging love, making up for my selfishness, my human condition. A warm feeling rushed over me as I invited PaPa back into this void that had been there for so long. In that moment, I heard the familiar voice say with a smile I could never deserve on my own, "Welcome home, my child."

The Fathers Story

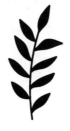

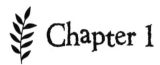

Chapter 1

Staring at the ceiling as I lay on my childhood bed, I swiped right on all the memories of high school and how I was the big fish in a little pond. Along the way, I ran into the ones of me laying on this very bed, hiding from all the yelling and things being thrown. In my mind, I was cringing under the covers all over again, trying to act as if I were asleep, in case they came in my room. I hated coming home for the holidays, having to go back and forth from my mom's new family and dad's family, for which he left Mom and me. I smiled, going in Dad's door, but the hate inside me grew with every opening of it to see this family that wasn't supposed to be. Don't worry, though. I was good at shoving it down. I learned it from my mom. I had watched her put up with Dad's verbal and eventual physical abuse as she would see me over his shoulder, smiling, then winking as if it were nothing. Afterward, she would tell me how God had a plan, how all this would turn out for good. Well, I'm still waiting on that.

Her new husband is a great guy. Kinda wish she would

have started off with him, not getting knocked up and marrying the first man who would take her. I don't really remember it, but I remember what came of it, this life of having no place, nothing stable. The day Dad left is still fresh in my mind. My mom was finally tired of it all and stood up to him, giving him the choice of us or that other woman. At this fight, I was now sixteen years old and a lot bigger with my growth spurt, so I went out to stand between them as a guard from further abuse. The look in his eyes was like the devil, since he had given in to him with another drinking bender. Staring me up and down, knowing this time he was no match, he grabbed his coat and slammed the door. The little boy in me was running out that door after him, but that little boy had to grow up and take care of his mom. She instantly changed from a strong woman into a broken one as she put her head in my chest, crying without control. This only resolved even more in me that I was never going to put anyone in this position. I'd just live my life and not invite someone else in.

My mom called me out of my memories, letting me know dinner was ready. I sat up looking one more time at all the posters covering holes I had punched in the wall, the ones I thought she hadn't found out about yet. I felt that little boy rising up again, so I reached into my pocket for one more pill so I could keep it all together, at least till I got back to school, where everything was different, where I was the main character in my story, the one I built where no one who could come in a destroy it.

Taking a deep breath, I came out of my room with an award-winning smile that kept all those I loved safe, because if they really knew this broken and angry person I was, it would destroy everything I had built.

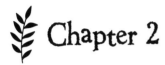 Chapter 2

The laughter was flowing freely around the holiday table, with my mom making moments like these my happy place when I was angry. I saved all that anger for the field, where I had finally found a place to take all this anger and let it loose, at the same time making a name for myself on a football field. I was a hyper kid, which made my dad crazy. Not knowing what to do with me, he put me in a junior league for football, which is where I found my place of therapy. I could just picture all that I hated and destroy it over and over and over again.

My parents had taken me to psychiatrists to see why I was so angry, but it didn't help, because when he questioned my parents as to my home life, it would be painted like the perfect American family. They were good at that. We went to church every Sunday as my parents became this fairy tale of how they met in college and my dad became the hero of the story, taking us both in. We sat there in those hard pews, hearing the gibberish about a perfect father in heaven who loved me so much that He sent his one and only son to set me free. That made no sense, because I was in this prison with no hope of parole.

See, this didn't seem possible to me, because my biological dad had gotten my mom pregnant while she was in college. It was a onetime thing; this jerk just came in with words that swept her off her feet, telling her all that any women wanted to hear. I think he was a football star too. I'm not really sure; we just don't talk about that part of life, since we had enough of a disappointment in my second dad. All I know is this God they spoke of sounded just like him, because I couldn't see either one of them.

The only time I felt free was on that field, mowing down whatever was in front of me. There I was in control. There I was the one dealing out the blows. There I was king. I remember the first time on the field, where I made that winning tackle, sending the crowd into a frenzy. It was like all my dreams coming true at once. All the recognition I was craving, actually needing, was there in such abundance, it overwhelmed me. I was where I wanted to always be. That moment set me up for what I wanted to do with my life. I mean, it's the only place I could take my anger and get recognition instead of another psychiatrist. Plus, if I made it, I could give my mom all that she deserved.

In middle school, I towered over the rest of the students, making everybody look up at me. With that came the respect I was always looking for. The coaches took me under their wings, giving direction and discipline. I never worked so hard on anything else, listening to every word they said, making them my parents, since they were more organized than my own.

There was one coach in particular who made an impact on my life, Coach Mills. As much as he pushed me on the field at the same time, his office door was always open. I could come to him with anything, knowing he was listening while at the same time actually caring about what I was going through. From time to time, he would offer to pray with me, and I just let him out of respect. Yet when he prayed, it was like whoever he was talking to was right there in the room with us. Afterward, I would always have a sense of peace I couldn't explain. It was like all my anger was gone. But then, I would get closer to home, and there it was again. Just like now. I could feel it growing inside me, but that's okay. I will just save it for the field.

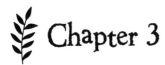

Chapter 3

The smiles had worn out on everyone, those smiles that kept the newest guest called awkwardness away. Now it was sitting at the head of the table. I smiled politely, covering the anxiety hidden behind this charade I put on every time I came home, initiating what the whole table wanted to do. Like the first guy who jumps in the pool on a hot summer day, just doing what they were all thinking of anyways. I went back to my room so I could pack up to go back to the fraternity house on campus. I was a shoo-in for this place with my strong athletic record and my position on the college football team. Laughing as I packed lifted the pressure I always felt when I came home. Behind the smile, I was remembering the fun I had with my frat brothers and how I found a dysfunctional family in them that wasn't trying to hide it. In fact, we relished in it by being all we could be on the field and larger than life off it.

Putting in the last bit of clothes, I heard my mom knock on the open door to my childhood room. She was wearing her perfect smile. As much as I hated being here, she could always make her little boy, the one she saw in her eyes, grin, no matter the situation. I could see the longing for me to stay as she glided in trying to hug me, and even though I resisted, just like fire meeting ice, I melted into her arms. What she didn't see was the tears welling up in my eyes in this melting process, but I quickly shut it down because I didn't want her to hurt. Maybe I just didn't want to let it go because I would fall apart on my childhood floor.

I backed away from her when I saw that my stepdad was suddenly lingering in the doorway. My stepdad stood there with his award-winning smile that allowed anyone to let their guard down. I just looked at him for a few seconds as I stood on the edge of an honest moment, where I would jump into his arms as if all the other disappointments called fathers never existed, but they did. I reached out, shaking his hand, leaving space between us but mostly because I respected him and how he took care of my mom and me in the last years.

Then it came, the Jesus huddle, where he pulled me in and my mom came from behind, holding me in their embrace, leaving me helpless. It's not as though I couldn't have taken both of them out, but they had a love for me that was more powerful than I could ever be. Mom started to pray over me while I just stood there, helpless. With her head laying sideways on my back, her voice sent a vibration through my whole body, right down to my soul. Slowly, that feeling of vulnerability started to take over, but I tackled it just like I did my opponents on the field. Still, there was a peace I had, which I could never explain, which I could never get from my pills. It reminded me of Coach Mills.

"Oh yeah, I gotta go see Coach Mills," I thought out loud, so they let me go even though they didn't want to.

I smiled, picking up my bag and giving one more hug to my hero, my mom. I looked her in the eyes one more time, wondering where this confidence came from, this unshakable faith that stared at me over the shoulder of my yelling stepdad, the hope that looked up at me with tears in them, telling me "It's going to be okay because God's got us." I just smiled and shook my head, quickly heading to the door. Jumping in the car, I got on this straight shot just outside the subdivision they lived in. My foot pressed hard onto the floor, trying to get away from all those memories and at the same time trying to catch a youth I could never have.

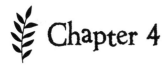

Chapter 4

The road to Coach Mills was on the way out of town, so I always made it a point to stop on my way back to college, which was about an hour away. Pulling into the driveway, I saw a bunch of cars there, a lot more than the usual ones. Knowing it was the holidays, I didn't think about it. I parked out in the yard, starting toward the door, swerving in and out of cars. I began to see that a lot of the license plates were from all over the United States, which gave me an eerie feeling. My pace sped up as I made the front door my only thought, like the goal line on a football field. I quickly maneuvered forward.

I stood at the front door, not wanting to ring the doorbell because that feeling was telling me something wasn't right. As I was about to knock, the coach's wife opened the door. Mrs. Mills stood wearing dress clothes with a mixture of sadness and smiles. Her arms penetrated the space between us like my mom did that day my dad ran out on us. I just stood there like a fencepost, not knowing what to do. It's not as if she had never done this before. Every time I came over, she was the first one at the door, looking at me as if she had been waiting since the last day I left. Mustering up the words, I asked, "What's the matter? Where's Coach?"

Her head lifted off my shoulders up to my ear, softly saying, "I'm sorry, Corey. He's gone. He died last night."

Rage took me by surprise as I pulled back, almost yelling at her, "What do you mean he is gone? No, no, no!"

She tried to console me, but none of that was happening. The one person who had been there no matter what, the one man in my life I could trust to be there, was not there anymore. The man who was immortal in my eyes was no longer. Mrs. Mills tried to hold me, but I just pushed her off, shaking my head as if I could make all this go away, like a bad song stuck in my head. Crazy laughter scattered out of my mouth as I walked backward, tripping over the gnomes I always made fun of when I came over. Falling to the ground, I crawled away as if some horrifying figure had just appeared in front of me, and I didn't know anything to do but run. So that's what I did.

The same intensity I had used to get to that front door was now carrying me back to my car. Mrs. Mills' voice carried through the cold air, trying to pull me back, but her words were drowned out by the first words she said: "He's gone." I tore out of the yard, getting on the interstate that led to school. Faster and faster, I went down this dark, cold road, trying to go just the right speed, like the DeLorean in *Back to the Future*. Trying to change time, trying to make these words go away, and trying to bring back this one hope that there was still something good in this world.

I rolled down the windows, letting the cold air hit my face just to feel, because I was so numb. With the radio up all the way, I drove that hour-long trip in what seemed like only a few minutes, because next thing I knew, I was pulling up to my fraternity, where cars were on the lawn, just like Coach's but for a different reason. I heard from my still-rolled-down window my name being yelled out from the front porch and these voices I ran to and not from, because I just wanted to become more numb.

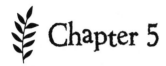

Chapter 5

Before getting out of the car, I reached in my pocket, pulling out my bottle of pills and pouring out a generous amount. After popping them in my mouth, I jumped out of the car, looking at my brothers on the porch. I lifted my arms in the air, giving out a yell that shook the ears of everyone within range. As I headed up to the guy waiting on me with a shot in his hand, I felt my phone vibrating in my pocket. Pulling it out, I saw it was my mom. Apparently, she had tried to call multiple times during my drive, but I missed them. I didn't want to talk to her anyway. With all these calls, I was guessing Mrs. Mills had called her. I just needed to forget, to get in that party and step out of this reality I couldn't comprehend.

All my brothers returned my war cry as I walked up the porch stairs. I grabbed the shot out of there hand, drinking it down. Then we all walked in with arms around each other's shoulders, giving out the same chant we gave on the field. The lights distracted my senses as I went around the room in a euphoric state since the pills were kicking in now. Bouncing back and forth from place to place, I continued my resolve to forget one shot at a time. I don't know how much time passed, but the partying had caught up with me, and I started feeling nauseated, so I stepped out on to the back porch to get out from under the crowd of smoke and lights.

Standing at the edge of the back porch, the music was fading from my ears as they closed the door at the same time I was following suit, as my senses were nonexistent. I just stared out into the backyard at all these people I didn't even know, carrying on like what had just happened to me didn't matter, kinda like the world did anyways, as I slowly died inside. I smiled a little as I relived the good moments with Coach. Honestly, they were all good. The laughter of him and Mrs. Mills danced around in my head as I chuckled a little more. Then the feeling that someone was watching me took over. Peeking out the corner of my eye, I saw two giggly girls looking over at me. My pride welled up, and my chest puffed out a little. Then I felt someone run into me, knocking me out of the elevated status in my head.

"What the hell?" came flying out of my mouth, but that quickly changed when I saw this little picture of innocence standing beside me now. Her eyes were the deepest blue, and she had on a little flowered summer dress. In my faded state, she glowed like an angel, an angel sent to rescue me from all that was going on in my life.

We talked for hours. I think it was, anyway. The whole night was coming to an end as my tolerance was past its limit, but my heart was restless, and she was my answer, at least for the night. I remember patches of making out, then heading back to my room. Then she was gone.

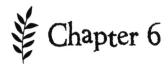

Chapter 6

School started up again, and life went back to normal. I was just sitting in class all day, waiting to get back on that field, where I was in control, where I didn't need to learn anything and I was in control. I was never really good at books because I could never sit still long enough to hear anything the teacher was saying. The only reason I got to college was from the football scholarship that Coach Mills helped me get.

Coach Mills. Man, I miss that guy so much.

I was awakened from the daydream by the bell, letting me know what I wanted was here. Grabbing my backpack, I tore off through the campus, straight to the locker room. I was always the first one there and the last one to leave. I never complained about all the extra practices on and offseason. Nothing in my life mattered to me as much as football. No matter how my life was, football was always the same, consistently there.

Tim came in after me into the locker room, giving me the same life-giving smile my stepdad gave. This confident guy was the most straight-up person I knew.

The only thing I didn't like was how he was always trying to get me to go to his Christian student meetings. I went a couple of times, but the whole singing and arm-waving thing freaked me out. Yet there was something about them. They never acted like they had it all together and life was perfect. Well, a few did. The rest of them would meet me where I was at. They kinda reminded me of the Jesus huddle my parents always did when I went home.

Tim gave me a slap on the shoulder, asking about how Christmas break had gone. We named him Timmy T because his last name started with a T, and it just seemed to fit his homely character. I just gave the scripted answers to keep him close enough to talk but far enough away not to get inside, like a passing neighbor you don't want to come in, so you just politely wave and run back inside. Still, he had this uncanny way of knowing if I was full of it or not. Sitting beside me, he put his arm around me, letting me know anytime I wanted to talk, I could call on him. Talking like guys do, facing forward, I looked at the floor, sheepishly nodded my head, and smiled.

As I was changing, I looked at my phone to see a text from the girl at the party I hooked up with. I knew that because I put flower dress on the description of her caller ID. That's how I keep them all straight, because there were so many. So many stories but no good ones. I hit the phone symbol in the top corner. Surprisingly, she answered pretty quickly, with her chipper voice that I liked so much. We talked for a minute, with the usual beginnings. Hearing that she was in a running car, I asked the flower dress girl where she was. Then, seamlessly, the conversation moved into the fact that she was at a doctor's office. Not really caring, I politely asked what was going on. Then came the talk that reached through the phone and punched me right in the chest.

All I remember is "I'm pregnant." There was a long pause as the flashbang wore off and I jumped straight into defense.

"Well, who else have you been with? Are you sure it's mine?" came flying out of my mouth like bullets shot at an intruder who threw this flash bang of a conversation. She tried to calm me down, but I was having none of that. She started to fire back at me with her own words, and instead of trying to figure this out, I did what I always did: run. I slammed the phone down, ending the conversation. Afterward, I just sat there shaking my head while Timmy T looked back at me with concern, but before he could ask, I grabbed my gear and headed to the field.

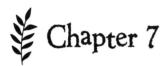

Chapter 7

My defensive coach, Coach Blake, was impressed with the intensity that I showed on the field that day. I plowed through the line like a pissed-off bull going after the red cape. All I could see was red anyway. I didn't know if I was mad at her for getting pregnant, at me for not being more responsible, at Coach Mills for leaving me, at my dad for being a jerk, or at God for letting this happen. The rest of the practice was a blur, and the hope I had of leaving it all on the field didn't even come near to being true. I ran and ran and ran just like I did that night not long ago from that truth I'm still running from. Yet it wasn't far enough.

I dressed down and just skipped the shower so I could get out of there. Tim reached out, grabbing my arm as I rushed out to show his concern.

"Slow down, William!" Tim urged, but I just pulled off, giving him a look that said he better back off. Still inside, I wanted to tell him everything, because if all this kept building up, I was going to explode. Slamming through the double doors sent a message to the rest of the team that I was not someone they wanted to approach right then.

I jumped into my car, speeding off to get to my room so I wouldn't have to look at anyone. As I drove, the people in the cars passing me seemed to look at me like they knew what a jerk I was. It was as if their thoughts of me jumped into my passenger seat, then onto my chest. I started having trouble breathing, and I could tell this was going to be a bad one this time. I'd had panic attacks for so long, but they steadily seemed to get worse and more frequent. At the next stoplight, I popped more relief from my bottle of Xanax, chewing them up so they would kick in faster. At least I think that worked. Really, I didn't care. I just wanted to keep my heart from beating out of my chest.

I think I took them just in time before I passed out, and when that familiar wave of relief came over me, all my cares faded away. I loved that first moment when they kicked in, because you could have slapped me and it wouldn't have made a difference. Now, at a slower pace, I smiled at my frat brothers as I strolled up to my room. Closing the door, I lay on my bed, finally relaxing. Then I thought the cops were at the door to serve the warrant for all my sins. I rushed up to the answer only to see her, the flower dress girl, and she was pissed. Her conversation started where I had ended it by hanging up on her.

She let me have it, and every word I tried to add in was quickly shut down. All her words were so fast I couldn't make sense of them, but the one sentence I did understand was "Well, you're the father."

That was it. I wasn't gonna take this crap from anybody, so I shot back, "The kid's not mine. It's your fault."

And that ended it. We stood there in silence as I waited for her reply, but I could tell that I had crushed her. Then the shame I felt started to take over, so I just slammed the door in her face. I stood in front of that closed door, listening to see if she had left, and then I heard the slow pace of her shoes fade down the hall. I went back to my bed to fall into it, because I had nothing left to give. As I was fading out, I heard Tim's voice in my head, telling me to talk to him. I mumbled back to the thought, "Okay." Then I passed out.

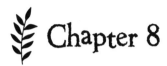

Chapter 8

I woke up later that day glad all this was over, or at least out of view. I lay there a few more minutes getting my bearings when, in the process, I came back to the thought I answered before I passed out to call Tim. I fumbled with my phone, trying to call before I thought about it too long, because if I did there were a million reasons not to but only one good reason to do it. The phone didn't even ring one whole time before I heard Tim's voice on the other end. I started just emptying out this graveyard inside my soul. I almost felt sorry for him, but his presence on the other end of that phone never tried to fix it or run out on me; it just listened.

I don't know how long I rambled, but by the time it was over, I was exhausted. There was a moment of silence as Tim allowed anything else that needed to be said. Then he responded with words that were so truthful, telling me he couldn't even imagine what I was going through but that he wanted me to know he was there no matter what. He started to encourage me to find the flower dress girl and make things right. I came back with reasons not to, but all of a sudden, I had an epiphany. I was just like my biological dad: the jerk who took off, the jerk who cared only for himself, the jerk I never wanted to be.

Tim offered to come over and pick me up to go and find her. He was afraid she might do something she might regret. That thought never crossed my mind, because I only had me on my mind. This was a new feeling of letting someone else inside this heart I had shut up for so long, this new discovery that the epiphany revealed encapsulated me, and I quickly agreed.

Tim met me at the front of the fraternity, and we started the search. I called everyone I knew, trying to trace back to who she was and where she lived. As we made our way through the campus, pieces of the puzzle came together, and we found out that she drove some hooptie and lived in some apartments off-campus. We raced off to go and find her, but when we got there, her car was gone. Just in case, I went and knocked on the door, but no one was there.

Heading back to Tim's car, I guess he saw the look of confusion and desperation spread all over my face. Sitting back in the passenger seat, I let out a sigh that said I was out of answers. Reading in on that, he suggested we pray. I was so lost right now, I had no fight in me to say no. He put his hand on my shoulder, bowing his head as I just stayed leaned back. When he started to speak that familiar peace from Coach Mills office came into that car. Listening to his words, I heard an intimacy that was undeniable, with a surety that someone else was there listening, caring, and always there, kinda like Coach Mills believed. I just stayed in that moment, enjoying the peace.

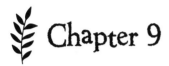

Chapter 9

When the prayer was over, he didn't talk about it but just started driving. Curious, I asked where he was going, and he just said he had a feeling. There was this clinic that all the guys knew from campus that took care of unwanted pregnancies. The facility was a landmark no one really talked about, because it had been there since abortion became legal. I heard a few stories of people who went there, but that was not a comfortable subject, so no one really talked freely about it. I started to get a sick feeling in my stomach as we got closer, not knowing that was the destination Tim was headed to. We slowed down, and as I looked out the window, I saw the flowered dress. I jumped up and put my hand on Tim's shoulder to get him to stop.

My surroundings that was just a moment ago a blur were now coming into focus. I knew it was the girl from the party because she was wearing the same dress she was wearing the night I meet her. She was sitting on a park bench right outside the clinic with an older lady who seemed familiar, but I just shrugged that thought off and focused back on the flower dress girl. Tim came to a stop, and I jumped out to go to her. Running up, I stopped in front of her, not knowing what to do. We just stared at each other for what seemed like forever. I could see the waterfall flowing down her rosy cheeks, with a look of regret. That's when I felt something forming in my eyes. It was a tear. The first one that fell gave permission for the rest of them to come out behind it.

She stood up and buried her head into my chest, sobbing uncontrollably. I just stood there and held her like I did my mom that day dad left us. As I held her, I looked over at the lady she was sitting with and saw her crying as well. Then it came to me who she was. It was Mrs. Mills.

What is she doing here? What's going on here?

Confused, I just stood there until the flower dress girl was through using my chest as a pillow to cry in.

"Mrs. Mills, what are you doing here?"

Leaning up from my chest, the flower dress girl said, "How do you know each other?"

Then the conversation of explanation came out. Apparently, Mrs. Mills had an abortion when she was younger. That's why she couldn't have kids of their own. That explained why Coach Mills always called me son. I never really questioned why they didn't have any kids. A few years after her abortion, Mrs. Mills sat on this bench and prayed for all the girls going in, offering a listening ear—not a protest or any sign of judgment. She had watched many girls go in there and helped a few. She had seen angry people with picket signs saying "God hates you" and "Turn back, you sinner." But Mrs. Mills was just there ready and willing to be whatever they needed and what they needed was someone who understood.

Tim came walking up and smiled as he gave Mrs. Mills a hug; apparently, she was pretty famous for what she did around the Christian community. We all sat down, starting a conversation to put the pieces together. There were tears and laughter as we became a weird little family on a park bench on a Tuesday.

Then I looked at the flower dress girl and said, "Hi."

She replied, "Hi."

Then the healing began.

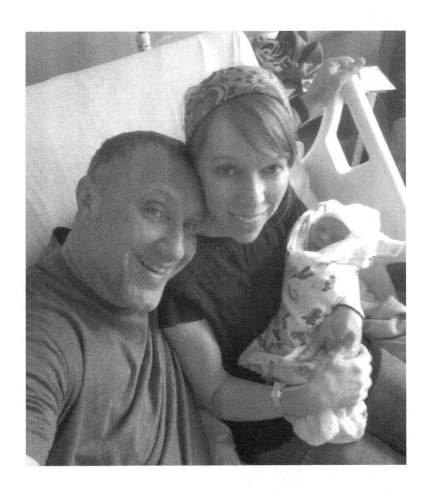

Me and my wife, and our newly adopted child.